Your A
Sexuality For Seniors

15 Simple Steps to Increase Intimacy in Your Relationships

In this incredibly informative book, Randy Dickason and Reverend Jenny Dickason share the secrets of their amazing marriage in a way that makes it easy for anyone to enjoy the same results into their "golden years."

While there are many books available that focus on the mechanics of great sex, this book focuses on the role of great sex in building great relationships. As you will learn from reading this book, when you have amazing sex, combined with open, honest communication, then you will have fulfilling and passionate relationships.

The authors of this book are in a long-term, committed, monogamous, heterosexual marriage; however, these 15 steps can be practiced by anyone, regardless of their marital status or sexual orientation.

Pick up a copy of this life-changing book today and experience the ecstasy that comes from embracing and expanding your sexual power.

Your Amazing
Itty Bitty®
Sexuality for
Seniors Book

15 Simple Steps to
Increase Intimacy in Your Relationships

Randy Dickason and
Rev. Jenny Dickason

Published by Itty Bitty® Publishing
A subsidiary of S & P Productions, Inc.

Copyright © 2016 Randy Dickason

Printed in the United States of America

Itty Bitty® Publishing
311 Main Street, Suite D
El Segundo, CA 90245
(310) 640-8885

ISBN: 978-1-931191-76-0

This book is lovingly dedicated to all of the people from our past relationships from whom we learned so much and to all the couples who endeavor to raise the bar by showing the world how much they love and respect each other.

Stop by our Itty Bitty® website to find interesting blog entries regarding sexuality for seniors.

www.IttyBittyPublishing.com

Or visit

www.sexualityforseniors.com

Table of Contents

Introduction
Step 1.   Amazing Sex at Any Age
Step 2.   Sensuality Outside of the Bedroom
Step 3.   Good Communication and Great Sex
Step 4.   Building Mutual Trust
Step 5.   Overcoming Old Paradigms
Step 6.   Knowing What Feels Good
Step 7.   Healthy Lifestyle Habits
Step 8.   Be Adventurous
Step 9.   Romantic Date Nights
Step 10.   Practice, Practice, Practice
Step 11.   Dealing With Health Challenges
Step 12.   Sex Shops Are For Couples Now
Step 13.   Professional Intervention
Step 14.   Little Things Mean a Lot
Step 15.   Keeping Relationships Positive

Introduction

As a long-time married couple, we were surprised when people would ask us if we were newlyweds. When we would answer that we had been married over twenty years, many would tell us that we needed to share the secrets of our successful relationship with others.

Based on those suggestions, the idea for this book was born. We are pleased to share this information with you and hope that you will apply the lessons contained in this book to your own relationships.

Finally, please know that the term "seniors" is a relative term. We needed to differentiate this book from the typical self-help books that are targeted to a younger audience. As you will see as you read this book, we believe you are as young as you feel.

Step 1
Amazing Sex at Any Age

You can have amazing sex at any age. Too often, couples buy into a misguided belief that as they age their sex lives will become boring, routine, infrequent, or non-existent. Following the steps in this book will show you that those misguided beliefs do not need to be your reality.

1. In good relationships, couples can come to recognize that amazing sex within the context of a loving relationship can be far more gratifying than "technically correct" sex.
2. Many younger couples focus on the quantity of sex rather than the quality of sex. Mature couples can come to the realization that quality sexual interactions can be far more rewarding than frequent sexual interactions that are lacking in a genuine intimate engagement.
3. Doing your research – whether through internet searches, or reading sexually-oriented books or manuals can contribute greatly to learning what couples can do to improve their sex lives. However, do not believe everything you read.
4. As you age, changes in your body *may* lead to your having amazing sex.

Positive and Negative Influences

There are many factors that can influence the quality of your sexual encounters. Some of the positive influences may include, but are not limited to:

Personal Issues
- Good personal hygiene
- Proper grooming
- Wearing attractive attire
- Willingness to laugh or smile

Environmental Issues
- Maintaining a warm home environment
- Creating a romantic bedroom setting
- Minimizing stress in the household
- Taking advantage of outside climate
  - Open windows for cool breezes
  - Go for natural lighting
  - Listen to the sounds of nature such as trees rustling and/or raindrops falling

Avoiding negative influences such as:
- Anger
- Negative judgment
- Refusing to let go of old stuff
- Allowing others to bring their negative energy into your household or your relationships

Step 2
Sensuality Outside of the Bedroom

"Sex Begins in the Kitchen"
Dr. Kevin Leman

Happy couples know that sensuality is not limited to the bedroom. Sensuality can be shared throughout the day… in any room in the house.

1.   Sensuality begins with your thoughts.
2.   Your sensual thoughts can be expressed with kind words.
3.   Kind, thoughtful words can lead to positive, sensual interactions.
4.   Partners in successful relationships have usually come to understand what is important and meaningful to each other.
5.   You don't have to agree, understand, or even necessarily *feel* what your partner feels to be responsive and supportive of your partner.
6.   Men, if you doubt the wisdom in this step, just ask your partner how she feels when she sees you washing dishes.

Shared Intimate Experiences
Outside the Bedroom

In Step 14 we will share more information about how "little things mean a lot." For now, here are some things you can do to share intimacy outside of the bedroom.

- Give tender touches.
- Give massages – neck, shoulders, hands, feet, full body.
- Buy flowers just because you care.
- Go to a coffee house to listen to live music.
- Present each other with small gifts.
- Hold hands while window shopping.
- Leave romantic notes for him/her.
- Regularly make thoughtful comments.
- Share loving gazes.
- Go outside at night and stargaze.
- Enjoy the sounds of a thunderstorm.

As you can see, non-sexual touch is very high on *this* list of intimate expressions. You may find that some, all or none of these are high on your list.

The real fun comes in finding intimate expressions that you can share with your partner.

Step 3
Good Communication and Great Sex

There is an old joke that goes, "what is a four letter word ending in 'k' that means intercourse." The surprise answer is "talk." This is perhaps the most important step in this book. The bottom line is that great sex begins with good communication.

1. Every relationship is about needs getting met.
2. Poor relationships are usually the result of one or both partners having unmet expectations.
3. Unmet expectations often lead to resentment. With respect to unmet expectations, in a troubled relationship it is common to hear one person say to the other, "You should have known how to make me happy." We call this the "psychic approach to communication."
4. It is incumbent upon each partner to be open, honest, clear and direct with respect to what his/her needs are and with respect to what his/her expectations are.
5. To the extent possible, each partner should endeavor to meet the needs of the other partner – whether those needs are sexual or non-sexual.
6. Good communication can continue to grow and develop over time – often over decades.

Keep it Simple

Couples should celebrate whenever they engage in good or great communications. Some of these communication celebrations may be the result of taking some "baby steps." At other times, there may have been major communication obstacles that have been overcome. In any event, never give up bettering the ways in which you verbally communicate.

Good communication can begin with three simple questions:
- What's working well in our relationship?
- What's not working well?
- What can I do to make our relationship better?

Probing questions to ask outside of the bedroom:
- What kind of day did you have?
- No matter what the answer, you can always ask, "How can I make it better?"

Probing questions to ask in the bedroom:
- What are you in the mood for? The answer could be anything from snuggling to role-playing the farmer's daughter and the traveling salesman!
- How can I help you relax or increase your enjoyment?

Step 4
Building Mutual Trust

Building mutual trust contributes immensely to couples having extraordinary sex. The dictionary offers numerous definitions of trust; however, we have found that the following things are essential to defining and/or building trust.

1. Expressing genuine, unconditional love.
2. Being willing to be vulnerable. When you really trust someone you do not have to "keep your guard up." You can be open and honest about your feelings.
3. Being secure enough in yourself to let go of concerns about your partner having close friendships (same or opposite sex) outside of your relationship.
4. Trusting your partner does not mean disclosing every single thing about your past relationships. It is okay to keep some things private when they do not have an impact on your current relationship.
5. Avoiding brutal honesty. When your partner asks, "Does this dress make me look fat?" The only acceptable answer is, "Why no, you look beautiful to me!"
6. Being consistent in what you say and how you act.

Letting Go

When there is a strong sense of mutual trust, you and your partner can really let go of fear, worry, self-doubt, etc., and experience truly mind-blowing sex. When you let go of preconceived expectations, sensuality can envelope every aspect of an encounter.

- Let go of fear and worry. Just go with the flow.
- Let go of the past, and disregard the future. Focus on being present in the moment.
- Let go of any sense of time when having a sensual encounter. Realize that in a trusting relationship each partner can be completely lost in moments of bliss.
- Recognize that deep trust does not occur overnight. Trust can develop and grow over weeks, months or years.

Understand that you may experience a wide array of feelings during the course of any relationship. When you stop trying to understand or categorize your feelings you will be better able to connect emotionally with your partner.

- Crying is okay.
- Allow time to process emotions.
- Be supportive – don't try to fix anything.

Step 5
Overcoming Old Paradigms

The greatest impediments to overcoming old paradigms are shyness and/or embarrassment. In particular, many couples are very hesitant to talk about their "private parts." Get over it!

1. If your partner trusts you enough (and has the courage) to ask questions about sensitive topics, you should be forthcoming with your answers.
2. When either or both of you engage in asking intimate questions and/or exploring "private parts," be willing to listen and learn. This advice applies to both sexes, but men often know less about female genitalia than women know about male genitalia.
3. Contrary to the old adage, an old dog *can* be taught new tricks. Be willing to learn about and try new things.
4. Be aware that what you don't know *can* hurt you – or at least have an adverse impact on your intimate relationships.
5. Explore each other's sexual fantasies, but know that having a fantasy does not mean that someone necessarily wants to act on it. It is perfectly okay to keep some fantasies to yourself.

Thinking Outside the Box

Once you release old paradigms, let go of religion-inspired inhibitions, and disregard social pressures regarding what is "right" or "wrong" in the bedroom, you can truly be free to enter a whole new world of sexual experiences.

- Start with the idea that sex does not *have* to be limited to the bedroom! Think Kevin Costner and Susan Sarandon in the movie "Bull Durham."
- Remember that having sex in a place that you normally don't can add to the excitement. Somebody thought about starting the Mile High Club!
- In the movie "Don Juan DeMarco," Johnny Depp sits across from a woman in a restaurant and, using her hand and fingers as surrogates, describes how he will make love to her. The sensuality blossoms into an explosion of ecstasy!
- Everyone has fantasies. Put your partner into one of your favorite fantasies and allow it to play out in your mind, enjoying the pleasures you will give and receive!
- Are there things you would like to try? Make a list and then start with one thing. Pretty soon you'll be adding to your list. Just sharing your lists with each other could be new, different and exciting!

Step 6
Knowing What Feels Good

"To know thyself is the beginning of wisdom."
Socrates

Once you "know yourself" you must be willing to share with your partner (in great detail) those things that feel good.

1. When asked, men tend to say that any genital contact feels good to them. Women, however, tend to be much more specific regarding what feels good since their sexual response is generally more complex than those of men.
2. As noted in Step 5, "Overcoming Old Paradigms," no area of your body should be considered "off limits." If it feels good, do it! (Of course, you should always ask first before "just doing it.")
3. Finally, if you are a Christian who has concerns about your "religious beliefs" and sexuality, just remember that in Hebrews 13:4 the Bible says, "Let marriage be held in honor among all, and let the marriage bed be undefiled." We believe this means that in the privacy of your bedroom, there is nothing to be ashamed of.

Special Touch Points

You can't expect your partner to find your "special touch points" if you don't know where they are yourself. In order to truly practice this step, you must put all embarrassment aside and masturbate – in private or together. Masturbation may involve the use of:

- Hands or fingers
- Vibrators (there are many varieties available for women or men)
- Dildos
- All of the above!

Once you know what really turns you on, you can share those discoveries with your partner! In addition to the typical "erogenous zones" here is a list of often overlooked touch points that can be stimulated with hands, lips, tongues, etc.:

- Ear lobes
- Toes and fingers
- Face and eyelids
- Creases in elbows and knees
- Thighs (inner and outer)
- Back of the neck
- Lower back

The only limitation is your own imagination!

Step 7
Healthy Lifestyle Habits

Overall good health can contribute significantly to having great sex; therefore, it is important to maintain a healthy lifestyle. Our friend Dianna Whitley writes in her Itty Bitty® Staying Young at Any Age Book that "the aging process is real, but it can be slowed down enormously, and some of it can even be reversed." Some things you can do to promote healthy living include:

1. Believing that it is never too late to begin taking care of yourself.
2. Doing everything in moderation.
3. Paying attention to your diet.
4. Including exercise in your daily routines.
5. Recognizing that rest and relaxation is important to maintaining good health.
6. Practicing healthy lifestyle choices with your partner!

Of course, you should always consult your doctor before undertaking any lifestyle changes. As they say in the advertisements for erectile dysfunction drugs, "Ask your doctor if your heart is healthy enough before having sex."

Finally, in Step 11, "Dealing With Health Challenges," we will discuss health challenges that some seniors may face.

Good Health Contributes to Great Sex

Sexual response can be a barometer for one's general health. You should always listen to your body and know when to seek medical help should you experience symptoms that concern you.

Habits/behaviors that contribute to good health:
- Eating organic foods whenever possible.
- Minimizing consumption of red meat.
- Eating lots of fresh fruits and vegetables.
- Staying fully hydrated.
- Establishing a daily exercise regimen.
- Getting plenty of sleep. (Naps are nice!)
- Practicing spirituality (meditation, prayer or yoga).
- Enjoying a cup of coffee/tea or an occasional alcoholic beverage.
- Making sure you include outlets for your creativity.

Habits/behaviors that contribute to poor health:
- Eating "junk food."
- Skipping your prescribed medications.
- Forgetting to brush and floss your teeth.
- Living a sedentary lifestyle.
- Worrying too much about trivial stuff.
- Engaging in addictive behaviors.
- Living with stress.
- Failing to cultivate supportive friendships.
- Having a negative attitude in general.

Step 8
Be Adventurous

Be bold and daring! Within legal bounds, and within your own sense of morality, there is nothing that spices up a relationship like new and exciting things to try. Some things to consider as you venture down this bold new path include, but are not limited to:

1. Be spontaneous… or not. Some men who take an erectile dysfunction (ED) drug may think spontaneity is out the door. "I need 30-45 minutes for the blue pill to kick in." Just know that sometimes the thrill of spontaneous erotic touch can overcome the need for an ED drug. And, if things don't respond "down there," it presents a wonderful opportunity for non-intercourse intimate engagement with your partner.

2. Consider viewing erotic videos together. There are many video producers that now focus on sensitive, romantic erotica where both partners appear to be enjoying themselves.

3. Where it is legal, be aware that medical marijuana can greatly enhance any sexual experience.

4. As long as it is mutual and not harmful, hurtful, or dangerous, be willing to try anything once.

For Your Consideration

Although most of your sexual encounters will be in your bedroom, there is nothing that says sex must only occur there. Here are some changes of venue for your consideration:

Sexual Encounters Outside the Bedroom
- In the shower or bathtub (Do not engage in intercourse in the water as that can irritate the vagina.)
- In the living room or den. (Be sure and close the blinds first!)
- In the kitchen. (Remember, as noted in Step 2, sex begins in the kitchen.)
- In your secluded backyard or patio. (Especially if the weather is nice!)
- In the guest bedroom. (Although not while guests are staying there!)

Sexual Encounters in New or Exciting Locations
- In hotels. There's just something about hotel sex that makes it exciting.
- While onboard a cruise ship. (In your private room of course.)
- While staying with friends or family. (There can be a thrill as you both try to do it quietly!)
- In your car. (While parked in a quiet, dark location.)

Step 9
Romantic Date Nights

It is important to schedule regular date nights. Couples that do this have learned that special date nights can keep things new and exciting. And, as a bonus, the excitement around date night can build throughout the day.

1. Remember what it felt like when you and your partner first began dating? You can recapture that feeling with date nights!
2. When you know that you will "get lucky" at the end of the date you can be playful all evening long.
3. Date nights can involve routine activities like dinner and a movie, or…
4. You can be open to experiencing new and adventurous dates, which include activities that are not normally part of your routine.
5. Always remember to include activities that appeal to both partners. If there are activities that one or the other partner is truly opposed to, then that should not be included as a date night activity.
6. For additional guidance on date night activities, please refer back to Step 2, "Sensuality Outside the Bedroom."

The Bedroom Environment

Once your date night activities move to the bedroom, it is important to pay attention to the bedroom environment.

Romantic bedroom environments might include:
- Soft lights
- Scented Candles
- Your favorite incense
- A gentle breeze from a fan
- Romantic music
- Erotic videos
- Scenic videos such as ocean waves or mountain vistas

The above are some of the more common environmental enhancements that seniors appreciate; however, don't be afraid to get creative in your approach.

Other stimulating environments might include:
- Strobe lights or normal room lights
- Sheets dusted with scented powder
- Protective bed covers so that you can spread flavored oils all over each other
- Very cool thermostat settings (Cool bedroom temperatures allow for a lot of snuggling under a blanket.)
- Open windows during a thunderstorm (The lightning flashes and thunder just might create a thrilling environment!)

Step 10
Practice, Practice, Practice

A fellow is walking through downtown Manhattan and he asks a stranger, "Excuse me, can you tell me how to get to Carnegie Hall?" With a totally straight face, the stranger answers, "Practice, practice, practice."

1. One night stands are for amateurs.
2. Sex gets better with years of practice.
3. Both partners should be willing to experience various types of orgasm.
4. Women, help your man to understand that there really is such a thing as an "afterglow" which both of you can experience.

There is an old Spanish saying, "para buen hambre, no hay pan duro." (For a good appetite there is no stale bread.) Some folks (men in particular) make a similar reference to sex implying that there is no such thing as bad sex. Well, at the risk of sounding sexist, we can definitely say that this does not hold true for most women. We are not suggesting that it's okay for one or the other partner to set unrealistic expectations; however, sometimes good enough is not really "good enough."

Be willing to go for the gold!

From Baby Steps to Giant Leaps

Most people are aware that women can be multi-orgasmic. Less known or discussed is the fact that both women and men can learn to experience multiple orgasms and/or multiple types of orgasms. As referenced in the bullet points for Step 5, "Overcoming Old Paradigms," when you "think outside the box" your understanding of orgasm can change. In fact, we have coined the phrase "poly-orgasmic" to refer to a variety of ways in which men and women can experience a whole new world of orgasms. A few of the types of orgasm you might experience are:

Orgasms specifically for women
- Clitoral and vulval orgasms
- Vaginal and g-spot orgasms
- Combined clitoral and g-spot orgasms

Orgasms specifically for men
- Penile orgasms
- Prostate orgasms

Orgasms for both
- Whole body orgasms
- Nipple orgasms ("nipplegasms")
- Anal orgasms (yes, there is such a thing)

Feel free to do your own research on this topic. You might be amazed at what you find!

Step 11
Dealing with Health Challenges

Health challenges need not end your sex life. They may result in your discovering more creative ways of exploring your sexuality. As noted in other steps, please consult your doctor when dealing with health challenges.

Some health challenges that seniors may face which can impact their sexual practices include:

1. Side effects from medications which can result in impotence, lethargy, loss of libido, etc.
2. Cancer, resulting in the removal of one or both breasts, cervix and/or uterus, prostate, and other body parts.
3. Benign prostate hypertrophy (BPH).
4. Urinary incontinence or urgency.
5. Delayed orgasm for either partner.
6. Orgasm with minimal ejaculation.
7. Ejaculation with minimal orgasm.

In Step 13, "Professional Intervention," we discuss some of the psychological aspects of dealing with sex-related problems. Be aware that not all medical doctors are trained to help couples deal with health issues that impact their sex lives. A therapist who specializes in sexual issues may be the best choice.

It's All Good

Whether health challenges are a result of a medical condition or simply from aging, they can compel couples to find new and exciting ways of experiencing their sexuality. Some of the ways of seeing sexuality "differently" include:

- Viewing sex as a mental experience.
- Viewing sex as a whole body experience.
- Viewing sex as a mind/body experience.
- Using sex toys as sex tools. (See below)
- Taking your time to engage and explore.
- Being responsible for your own orgasm.
- Recognizing that you can have very satisfactory sexual encounters even when "conventional sex" is not an option.

One of the best kept secrets with respect to male orgasm is that it is not necessary for a man to have an erection to have an orgasm. In fact, there is a massager that is designed to fit over the hand (with a couple of sets of springs) that allows a man to grip around his frenulum allowing him to have a unique orgasm.

And men, you can use this handy massager on your partner. She may need to show you the exact placement that she prefers, but even the demonstration can be a real turn on!

Step 12
Sex Shops Are For Couples Now

The old image of an "adult shop" or "sex shop" as a dark, dirty, smutty place where perverts hang out is a remnant from years past. Today's sex shops are very couple-friendly. Most of the sex shop workers that we have encountered are:

1. Knowledgeable experts in their craft.
2. Delighted to answer your questions.
3. Happy to direct you to the products that will best meet your needs.
4. Willing to respect your comfort level.
5. Pleased to have seniors as customers.
6. Proud of the service that they provide.

Many sex shops carry just about anything you can imagine. Regardless of your comfort level, in general they are an excellent place to learn about and/or purchase items that will truly enhance your sexual encounters. You may wish to start your exploring with the following areas of the shop:

1. Lotions, lubes and massage oils
2. Erotic books and videos
3. Sensual attire for women or men
4. Sex toys for men and women

Fun, Fun, Fun

Although some folks prefer the anonymity of ordering sex toys and other libido-enhancing items online, many prefer the fun and excitement of visiting their local sex shop, where they can ask questions of the expert staff and receive answers that are specific to their personal interests. Some of the items you may be interested in include:

- "How to" books and videos
- "Bullet style" vibrators
- G-spot and prostate vibrators
- Orgasm enhancing lubes and lotions
- Flavored (edible) massage oils
- Fancy or plain condoms

Most shops offer an array of seasonal items which can help you bring the thrill of your favorite holidays into your sexual encounters.

- Holiday decorations (New Year's Eve, Valentine's Day and St. Patrick's Day are their big sellers.)
- Costumes (Not just for special events!)
- Romantic and sexually explicit greeting cards. (One of their best sellers is a booklet of romantic gift certificates which you can give to each other.)

Your imagination and your preferences are the only limitations!

Step 13
Professional Intervention

"You don't have to be sick to get better."
Rev. Dr. Michael Beckwith

Sometimes, in spite of all of their best efforts, couples may encounter relationship and/or sexual challenges with which they need professional help. Professional intervention may include couples counseling, individual counseling, and in some instances, individual psychotherapy.

1. If possible, find a licensed therapist. Conduct a pre-interview to make sure that the therapist is a good fit for both you and your partner.
2. Consider visiting a self-help group or attending a workshop or seminar.
3. For some couples, spiritual counseling may be the best alternative. (Be sure the spiritual advisor is open-minded.)
4. Ignore most television and radio therapists. The fact is, they are first and foremost entertainers, not therapists.
5. Be aware that most therapists can quickly ascertain what the real problem is versus what you describe as the "presenting problem."

It's Okay to Ask For Help

Professional intervention can often help individuals and couples understand where some of their "sexual hang-ups" and relationship challenges come from. Once the roots of the problem are uncovered, real healing and personal growth can occur.

Many sexual problems can be the result of a strict religious upbringing which can cause feelings of:
- Shame
- Guilt
- Fear
- Extreme modesty

Other issues that counselors/therapists can help you overcome may include:
- A lack of self-love and poor self-image
- Negative body issues
- Issues from your childhood
- Relations with adult children or parents
- Stresses – financial, career, workload
- Addictions – alcohol, drugs, gambling

While friends can be part of a great support system, they should not be counted on to provide the appropriate guidance that couples may need when serious emotional issues come up. One of the most important things that a professional therapist provides is a detached, unemotional view of the situation.

Step 14
Little Things Mean a Lot

Kitty Kallen sang about this in her 1954 hit song "Little Things Mean a Lot." The message she shared then still holds true today.

1. Encourage and support your partner's dreams and ambitions.
2. Find hobbies and interests that you and your partner can share together.
3. Avoid stereotypical beliefs. (Many guys enjoy "chick flicks" and many gals enjoy sporting events, sci-fi or action movies.)
4. Say "I love you" often... and mean it!
5. Listen to your partner, and ask for feedback about being more affectionate.
6. Remember Step 2, "Sensuality Outside the Bedroom." Your expressions don't have to be overtly sexual to mean a lot to your partner.
7. Pay attention to how your partner responds to the little things you say and do. Those reactions can help you understand what you need to do more or less of.

On the following page we touch on some of the little things that you can do to show your partner how much you love him/her.

Simple Demonstrations of Intimacy

Many of the steps in this Itty Bitty® Book have dealt with sexual issues. While senior sexuality is the main theme of this book, in reality we believe that simple demonstrations of love, affection and respect are perhaps the most important part of enhancing intimacy in your relationships.

Little things you can do to show that you care:

- Buy flowers without having a reason.
- Touch your partner often (throughout the day) in non-sexual ways.
- Hold hands when crossing the street.
- Sit close together when dining out.
- Leave love notes for your partner.
- Always kiss goodbye or hello when leaving or returning to the house.
- Say "I'm sorry" when you mess up.
- Offer a shoulder to cry on.
- Tell your partner how much you enjoy spending time together.
- Give your partner a quick massage.
- Make frequent eye contact when speaking to your partner.

In the movie "The Way We Were," Katie tenderly reaches up to brush the hair from Hubbell's face. Reviewers often say it is one of the most passionate, romantic moments in movie history. And, it was not in the script!

Step 15
Keeping Relationships Positive

It is easy to focus on things that go wrong in a relationship. Avoid that temptation and always try to focus on the positive.

1. Shared spirituality can be a key part of any relationship.
2. Cultivate friendships with like-minded individuals.
3. Recognize that there is power in the words you use.
4. Offer praise, compliments, and words of appreciation at every opportunity.
5. Recognize that in every relationship – and in life in general – everything happens for a reason.
6. Avoid getting together with girl/guy friends and criticizing your partner.
7. Make lists of all the large and small positive things your partner does for you. Practice finding things to do together and occasionally do something that may be completely out of your comfort zone.

It has been said that people live up to what is expected from them. If you always affirm that your partner is a loving, caring, intelligent, considerate human being, you will be amazed at how quickly they become exactly that!

Re-read This Book with Your Partner

Each step in this Itty Bitty® Book can lead to deeper understandings of yourself, your partner, and your relationships with others around you.

By re-reading this book with your partner, you can open the door to exploring the most intimate aspects of your relationship. It is important to know that sexual response can be a barometer for other aspects of your relationship. Sexual ecstasy is usually an indication that other areas of your relationship are going well. Sexual dysfunctions, however, may be symptomatic of other problems in your relationship.

Some things you can do to make sure you are keeping your relationships positive include:

- Letting go of the small infractions.
- Shifting your focus from what is wrong to what is right.
- Regularly creating new and exciting shared experiences.

We believe that by practicing the steps outlined in this book, your relationships will flourish and grow in love and understanding. Having a great sex life enhances all other aspects of our lives and can help us look, feel and act younger!

We wish you abundant blessings, playfulness and joy on your journey!

You've finished. Before you go…

<u>Tweet/share that you finished this book.</u>

Please star rate this book.

Reviews are solid gold to writers. Please take a few minutes to give us some itty bitty feedback.

ABOUT THE AUTHORS

Randy Dickason is a human resources consultant with over 35 years of experience handling employee issues in the workplace. In addition to having extensive employee relations experience, Randy is a classically trained flutist and harmonica player. Randy also plays Native American flute and he believes in the healing power of music.

Reverend Jenny Dickason is a minister, personal chef, singer, writer, networking specialist and event planner. Jenny facilitated a spiritual and business networking meeting called the W.I.L.D. Women (Wonderful, Intelligent, Loving and Divine) Network for many years in Phoenix, AZ. Jenny also enjoys traveling whenever possible.

Together, Randy and Jenny have raised three daughters and they have both been actively involved in New Thought churches in Phoenix, Arizona.

If you enjoyed this Itty Bitty® Book you might also enjoy …

- **Your Amazing Itty Bitty® Have More Sex Book** – Jan Robinson

- **Your Amazing Itty Bitty® Staying Young At Any Age Book** – Dianna Whitley

- **Your Amazing Itty Bitty® Heal Your Body Book** – Patricia Garza Pinto

And many other Itty Bitty® Books available online.

Made in the USA
San Bernardino, CA
04 August 2019